AIR FRYER COOKBOOK FOR BEGINNERS
2021

Make Tastier, Crisper Food for You
and Your Family,
with Lots of Easy and Delicious Recipes
for Beginners.
Help Your Body Lose Weight by Eating.

Violet H.Scott

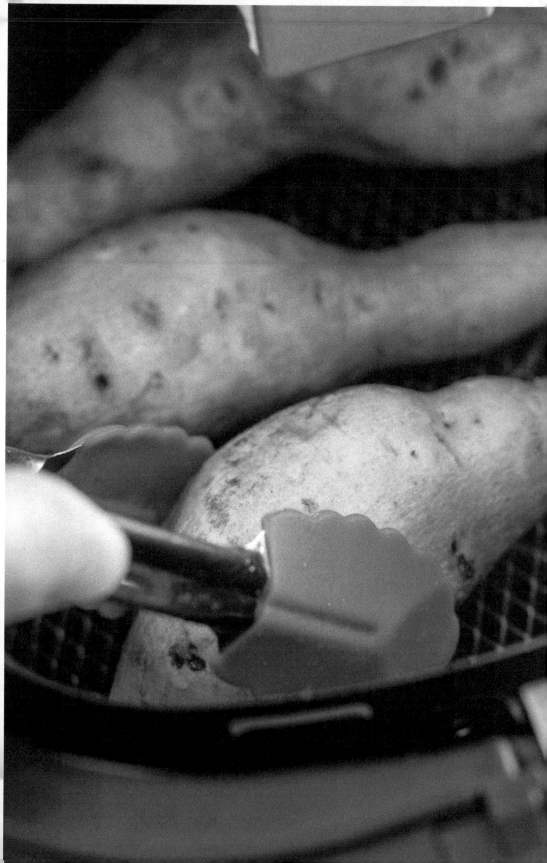

Table of Contents

Introduction 93

Recipes 94

Keto Airfryer Recipes

AIR FRYER BUTTER ZUCCHINI VEGETABLES

30 to 60 min

185 kcal

light

Portion size For 4 people

Ingredients

600 g yellow zucchini

 onion

2 Garlic cloves

1 Dossier spoon of olive oil

 salt

 pepper

70 g butter

Instructions

Wash and clean the zucchini and cut into bite-sized pieces of approx. 2 × 2 cm. Peel the onion and garlic, cut the onion into wedges, finely dice the garlic. Place in a bowl with the zucchini and mix with the oil. Salt and pepper.

Put the prepared ingredients in the cooking container with the paddle in place, add the butter and set the timer for 20 minutes. Start the device. If the vegetables are still too firm, simply extend the cooking time by a few minutes.

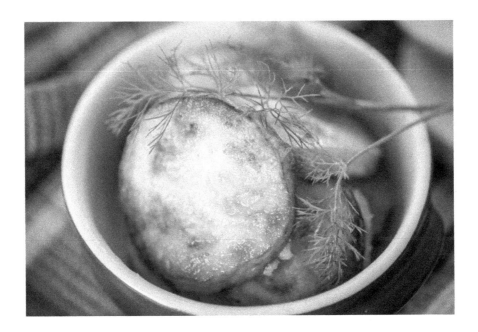

FAST TURKEY BURGERS RECIPE

Yield: 4

Prep time: 7 minutes

Cook time: 12 minutes

Total time: 19 minutes

Ingredients

1 lb. ground turkey

2 garlic cloves

3/4 tsp sea salt

1/2 tsp ground black pepper

1/2 tsp dried basil

1 Tbsp olive oil

Instructions

Preheat the air fryer to 360F for 5 minutes.

Combine the ground turkey, olive oil, minced garlic, sea salt, pepper, and dried basil in a bowl.

Divide the burger mix into 4 equal size balls and flatten them into patties.

Depending on which size of air fryer you have, you'll be able to make 2 or up to 4 air fryer turkey burgers at a time.

Cook the turkey burgers in the air fryer for a total of 12 minutes, flipping after 8 minutes, or until your desired degree of doneness.

If you're making burgers with cheese, add it after you flip the burgers.

Serve hot with your favorite burger toppings like bacon, lettuce, tomatoes, onion, pickles, or avocado slices.

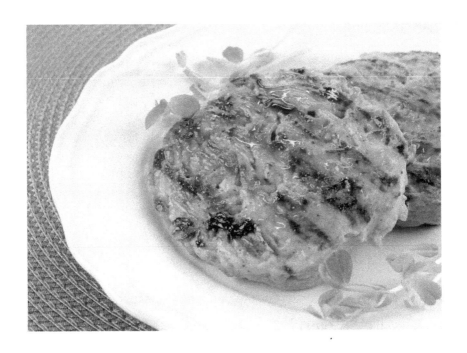

AIR FRYER CHEDDAR SCRAMBLED EGGS

Yield: 2 servings

Prep time 3 minutes

Cook time 9 minutes

Total time 12 minutes

Ingredients

1/3 tablespoon unsalted butter

2 eggs

2 tablespoons milk

salt and pepper to taste

1/8 cup cheddar cheese

Instructions

Place butter in an oven/air fryer-safe pan and place inside the air fryer.

Cook at 300 degrees until butter is melted, about 2 minutes.

Whisk together the eggs and milk, then add salt and pepper to taste.

Place eggs in pan and cook it on 300 degrees for 3 minutes, then push eggs to the inside of the pan to stir them around.

Cook for 2 more minutes then add cheddar cheese, stirring the eggs again.

Cook 2 more minutes.

Remove pan from the air fryer and enjoy them immediately.

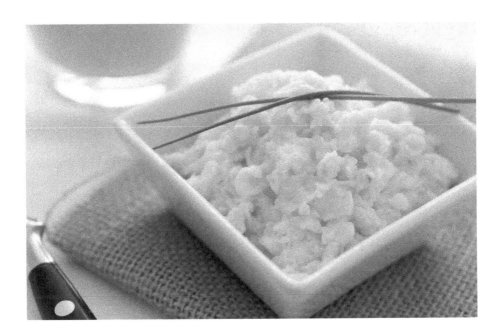

AIR FRYER SLICED HOT DOGS

Yield: 4 servings

Cook time

5 minutes

Total time

5 minutes

Ingredients

4 hot dogs

4 hot dog buns, sliced down the middle

Instructions

Preheat air fryer to 400 degrees.

Cook hot dogs for 4 minutes until cooked, moving basket once halfway through to rotate them.

Place hot dogs into hot dog buns.

Cook hot dogs in buns an additional 1-2 minutes, still at 400 degrees.

Enjoy immediately

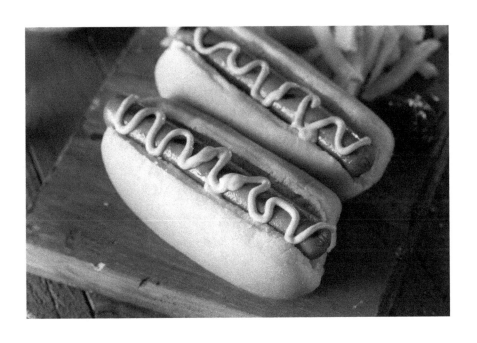

CRISPY BREAD & BACON

Yield: 4 servings

Cook time

8 minutes

Total time

8 minutes

Ingredients

7 ounces of bacon (approximately 8 slices)

1-2 pieces of bread

Instructions

Place 1-2 pieces of bread at the bottom of your air fryer underneath the basket. *

Put bacon in air fryer evenly in one layer. Cut bacon in half if too long.

Cook in air fryer at 350 degrees for 8-10 minutes, until it's at your desired crispiness. **

Enjoy immediately.

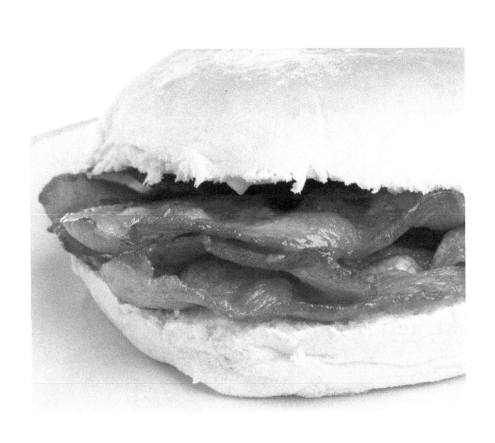

FAST AIR FRYER PORK CHOPS

Yield: 4 servings

Prep time

1 minute

Cook time

10 minutes

Total time

11 minutes

Ingredients

4 pork chops (boneless, bone-in, thin, or thick)

salt and pepper to taste

Instructions

Preheat air fryer to 400 degrees.

Season each pork chop with salt and pepper generously.

Place pork chops in the air fryer in a single layer.

Cook for 10-15 minutes*, flipping halfway through until the pork chops JUST hit 145 degrees at its thickest point.

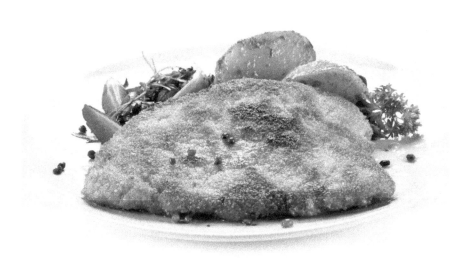

HEALTHY ROASTED CARROTS

YIELD: 4 SERVINGS

Prep time

5 minutes

Cook time

15 minutes

Total time

20 minutes

Ingredients

16 ounces of carrots

1 teaspoon oil

salt and pepper (to taste)

Instructions

Peel carrots and cut into 2-inch chunks. Cut any larger pieces in half to make all pieces a similar size.

Preheat air fryer to 360 degrees.

Toss carrots in about 1 teaspoon of oil. *

Place carrots in air fryer and cook for 15-18 minutes, shaking every few minutes.

Test carrots with a fork for tenderness. They are done when it glides through the carrot easily.

Add salt and pepper to taste and shake basket to coat.

Serve and enjoy immediate

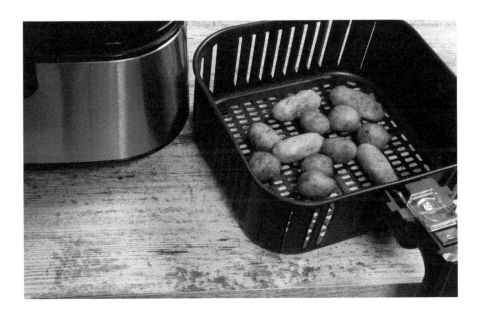

HEALTHY AIR FRYER BUFFALO CAULIFLOWER

Yield: 4 servings

Prep time

5 minutes

Cook time

11 minutes

Total time

16 minutes

Ingredients

1 head of cauliflower, cut into florets

1/4 cup buffalo sauce

Instructions

Preheat air fryer to 400 degrees.

Add cauliflower into the air fryer and cook for 7-8 minutes.

Remove cauliflower from the air fryer and place inside a bowl.

Add buffalo sauce to cauliflower and mix to coat cauliflower evenly.

Add the cauliflower back to the air fryer, turn temperature to 350 degrees, and cook for about 3 minutes.

Remove buffalo cauliflower from the air fryer and enjoy immediately.

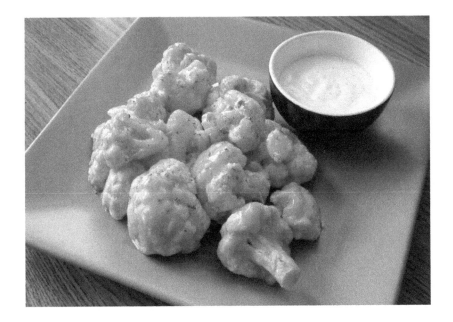

AIR FRYER BEEF HAMBURGERS

Yield: 4 hamburgers

Prep time

5 minutes

Cook time

8 minutes

Total time

13 minutes

Ingredients

1-pound ground beef, thawed (preferably 80/20)

1 clove garlic, minced

1/2 teaspoon salt

1/4 teaspoon pepper

Instructions

Preheat air fryer to 360 degrees.

Mix together the ground beef, minced garlic, salt, and pepper with your hands.

Form ground beef into 4 patties and press them down with the back of a pie plate to make them evenly flat.

Place hamburgers in a single layer inside the air fryer.

Cook for 8-12 minutes, flipping halfway through cooking for medium-well hamburgers. *

Carefully remove hamburgers from the air fryer, ** place onto hamburger buns (if using), and add desired toppings.

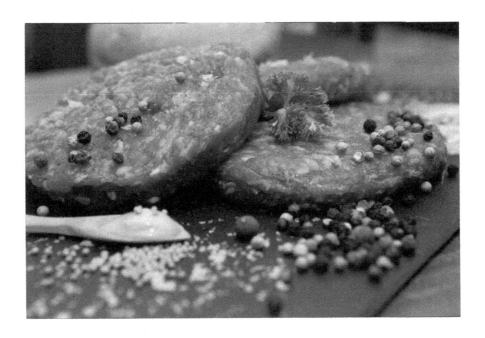

SALT & PEPPER BOILED EGGS

Yield: 4 servings

Ingredients

4 eggs

salt and pepper to taste

Instructions

Preheat air fryer to 270 degrees.

Place eggs in the air fryer, preferably on a wire rack, and cook for 15-17 minutes.

Immediately place eggs in a bowl full of cold water and ice until cool, at least 5 minutes.

Peel eggs and top with salt and pepper or refrigerate up to one week.

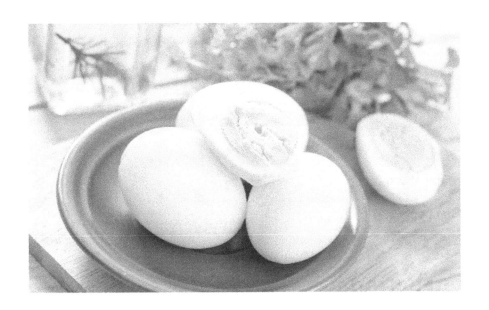

HAM & EGG CUPS (

Servings6 servings

Calories97kcal

Ingredients

6 slices prosciutto

6 eggs

1/2 cup baby spinach

1/4 tsp pepper, salt optional

Instructions

Air Fryer Egg Cups

Preheat your Air Fryer or Oven to 375.

While it preheats, lay one piece of prosciutto inside each cup, pressing to line the bottom and sides of each cup.

As long as your muffin tin is on the newer side, you do not need to spray the tin first – as the prosciutto cooks, it will naturally pull away from the tin as it cooks. If you're not sure, go ahead and spray or drizzle a little oil inside first.

Gently press about 4-5 spinach leaves into the bottom of each cup.

Crack one egg into each cup. Then just sprinkle with a little pepper and they're ready to go into the oven or air fryer.

Bake in the Air Fryer. Carefully transfer your muffin tin or muffin cups to the air fryer (leave a little space between them), and close. Cook for 10 minutes.

Bake in Oven: If using silicone muffin cups, set them on a baking sheet. Set the muffin tin or baking sheet on the middle rack and cook for 12-13 minutes for a medium-runny egg.

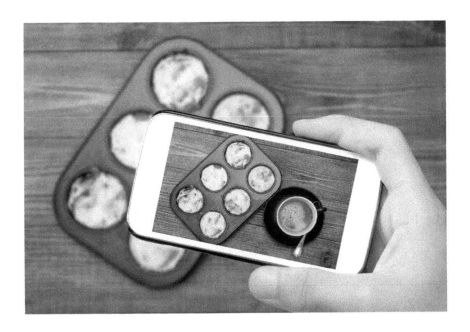

HEALTHY STEAK & CHICKEN KABOBS

Yield: 6 Servings prep time: 30 minutes cook time: 10 minutes total time: 40 minutes

Ingredients

2 Boneless Skinless Chicken Breasts

1/2 lb. Sirloin, or similar

1 Small Zucchini

1 Small Onion

1 Yellow Pepper

1 Green Pepper

Grape Tomatoes

2-3 tbsp Worcestershire Sauce

1 tsp Lemon Pepper

1/2 teaspoon Salt

1/4 tsp Black Pepper

8" Metal or Wood Skewers (Or however long your air fryer will hold.)

Instructions

Allow wooden skewers to soak for 10 minutes prior to cooking. Metal skewers do not need to soak. Rinse and slice all vegetables into 2" pieces.

Cut beef and chicken into 2" pieces. Add beef to a bowl and marinade with Worcestershire sauce, 1/2 teaspoon salt, and 1/4 teaspoon black pepper. Add chicken to a separate bowl and sprinkle with 1 teaspoon of lemon pepper.

Beginning with meat on each one, add beef and vegetables to skewers. Add chicken and vegetables to other skewers. Vegetables can be added in any order you like. Avoid adding steak and chicken to the same kabob due to different cook times.

Place kabobs in the air fryer basket in a single layer. Mine held 3 kabobs at a time. Cook in the air fryer at 400 degrees Fahrenheit for 9-10 minutes for chicken kabobs and 10-12 minutes for beef kabobs.

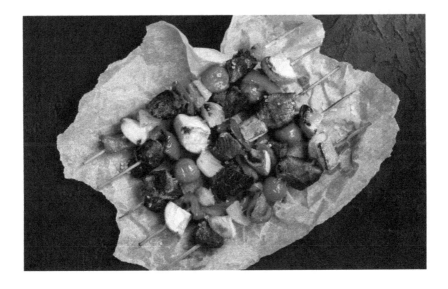

AIR FRYER TASTY SHISHITO PEPPERS

Prep Time: 5 minutes Cook Time: 4 minutes Total Time: 9 minutes
Servings: 4

Ingredients

½ lb. shishito peppers

1 tsp avocado oil or other oil with a high smoke point

Lemon Aioli

½ cup vegan mayonnaise, or your favorite mayo

2 tbsp lemon juice, freshly squeezed

1 clove garlic, finely minced

1 tbsp fresh parsley, finely chopped

¼ tsp each sea salt and pepper

Instructions

Combine all ingredients for the Lemon Aioli in a small bowl. Set aside to allow flavors to blend.

Preheat the air fryer to 390°F. for 3 minutes.

Toss shishito peppers with oil, then add to the basket of the air fryer in a single layer.

Fry for 4 minutes. Push pause and check for doneness. Peppers should be slightly softened and lightly blistered. If not done, cook for another minute or two.

Remove to a serving dish, squeeze a little fresh lemon juice overall and sprinkle with sea salt. Serve with Lemon Aioli.

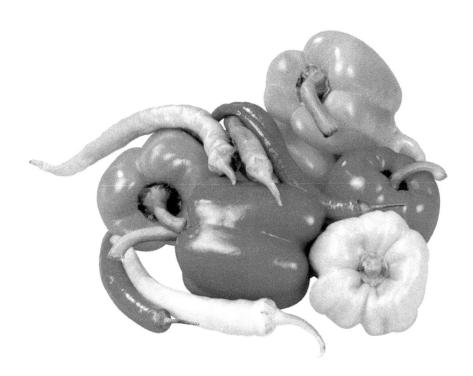

AIR FRYER BACON BRUSSELS SPROUTS

Prep Time: 5 minutes

Cook Time: 18 minutes

Total Time: 23 minutes

 Servings: 4

Ingredients

¾ to 1 lb Brussels sprouts

1 tsp olive oil

1 tsp balsamic vinegar

2 slices bacon, nitrate-free

1 pinch salt and pepper, to taste

Instructions

Wash and trim the Brussels sprouts first. Trim the tough stem end and remove any damaged leaves. Pat them dry.

Preheat your air fryer to 380°F. for 3 minutes

In a medium bowl, toss with oil and balsamic vinegar.

Cut bacon slices into one-inch pieces. Add the sprouts to the air fryer basket and top with the bacon pieces.

Air fry for 16 - 18 minutes, shaking the basket at least once partway through the cooking time.

Check for doneness with a fork and add a minute or two more frying time, if needed.

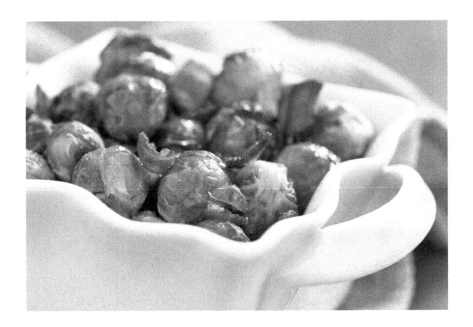

LOW CARB ZUCCHINI FRIES

Prep time

5 mins

Cook time

10 mins

Total time

15 mins

Servings 4

Ingredients

2 medium zucchinis

1 large egg beaten

⅓ cup almond flour

½ cup parmesan cheese grated

1 tsp Italian seasoning

½ tsp garlic powder

¼ tsp sea salt

¼ tsp black pepper

olive oil cooking spray

Instructions

Cut the zucchini in half and then into sticks about ½ inch thick and 3-4 inches long.

In a bowl, combine the almond flour, grated parmesan, Italian seasoning, garlic powder, sea salt, and black pepper. Mix to combine. Set aside.

In a separate bowl, whisk egg until beaten.

Dredge zucchini sticks in the egg wash and then roll and coat in the almond flour breading mixture. Place on a plate (for air fryer) or a lined baking sheet (for the oven).

Generously spray the zucchini sticks with olive oil cooking spray.

Air fryer Directions:

Working in small batches (depending on the air fryer size), place the zucchini fries in a single layer in the air fryer and air fry at 400°F (200°C) for 10 minutes or until crisp and golden.

Oven Directions:

Bake at 425°F (220°C) for 18-22 minutes, flipping them over halfway through until they are golden and crisp.

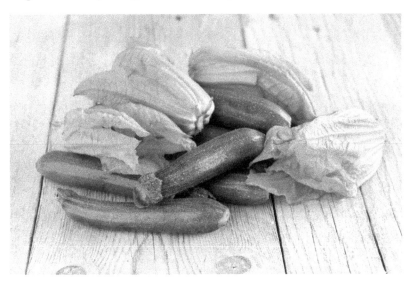

AIR FRYER RAMEKIN BAKED EGGS

Prep Time: 4 minutes

Cook Time: 16 minutes

Total Time: 20 minutes

Servings: 2

Ingredients

4 large Eggs

2 ounces Smoked gouda, chopped

Everything bagel seasoning

Salt and pepper to taste

EQUIPMENT

Air Fryer

Instructions

Spray the inside of each ramekin with cooking spray. Add 2 eggs to each ramekin, then add 1 ounce of chopped gouda to each. Salt and pepper to taste. Sprinkle your everything bagel seasoning on top of each ramekin (as much as you like).

Place each ramekin into the air fryer basket. Cook for 400F for 16 minutes, or until eggs are cooked through. Serve.

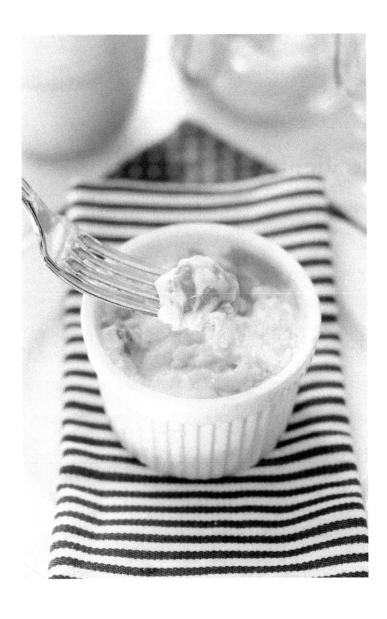

AIR FRYER BUNCH KALE

Cook time

9 minutes

Total time

9 minutes

Ingredients

1/2 bunch kale

Salt

Drizzle of olive oil

Instructions

Pre-heat the air fryer to 380.

Cut the kale from the stems, then cut that into small pieces.

Fill the bottom of a large pot about 1-inch high. Put in an expandable steamer basket.

Put the kale into the steamer basket and put the lid on the pot. Turn the heat up to high and let it steam for five minutes.

Remove the steamer basket from the pot.

Using a pair of tongs, move the kale pieces from the steamer basket to the air fryer basket.

Drizzle a tiny bit of oil (approximately 1 teaspoon or less) on the kale chips. Sprinkle them with salt.

Cook for two minutes, shake the air fryer basket, then cook for an additional two minutes.

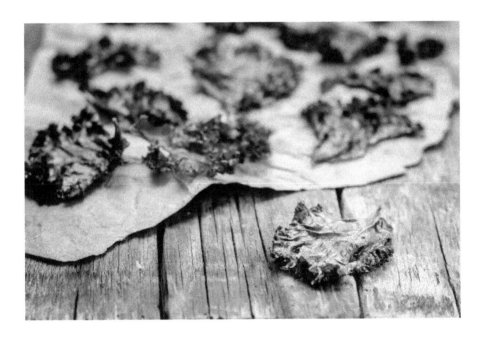

AIR FRYER RANCH JALAPENO POPPERS

Prep Time10 minutes

Cook Time10 minutes

Total Time20 minutes

Servings 4 servings

Ingredients

6 jalapenos halved and seeded

1 tbsp ranch dressing powder

4 ounces cream cheese softened

1/4 cup cheddar cheese shredded

1/4 cup green onion sliced finely

1 pound bacon

Instructions

1. Wash the jalapenos and cut them lengthwise, removing the seeds and membrane. Wear gloves if you have them

2. Combine the softened cream cheese, cheddar cheese, ranch powder, and green onions in a bowl, until well mixed.

3. Place 1-2 tbsp of filling in each jalapeno half, then wrap it in a slice of bacon.

4. Cook them in your air fryer at 400F for about 10 minutes or until the bacon is cooked and starting to crisp. Let cool and enjoy!

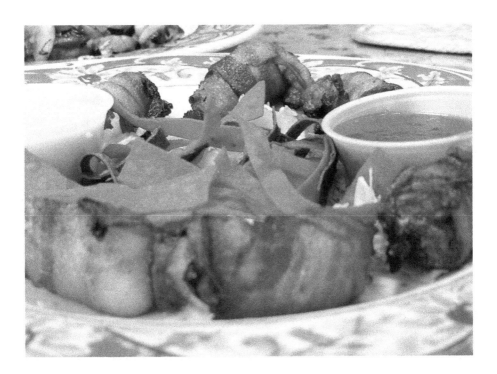

HEALTHY AIR FRYER TURKEY LEGS

Prep Time10 minutes

Cook Time21 minutes

Servings2

Ingredients

2 turkey legs

1 tbsp sea salt

1/2 tsp chili powder

1/2 tbsp garlic powder

1/2 tsp paprika

1/4 tsp basil

1/2 tbsp Old Bay

olive oil spray

Instructions

Preheat air fryer to 390 degrees F.

Mix together dry rub ingredients in a bowl. Rub on all sides of legs.

Spray inside of air fryer basket with olive oil spray and lay legs inside. Spray top of legs with olive oil spray.

Close drawer and cook at 390 degrees F for 21 minutes. Check at thickest part of leg to ensure internal temp. is 165 F. Remove from basket and allow to rest for 5 minutes before slicing meat off of bone and serving.

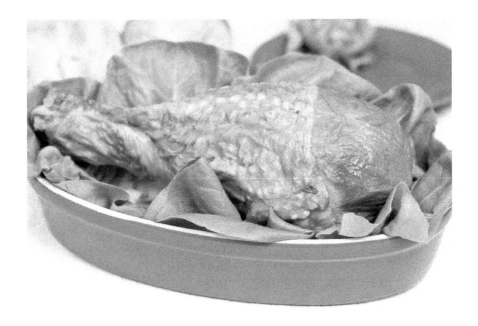

AIRYER LOW CARB SHRIMP SCAMPI

Prep Time: 5 minutes Cook Time: 10 minutes Total Time: 15 minutes

Servings: 4

Ingredients

4 tablespoons (4 tablespoons) Butter

1 tablespoon (1 tablespoon) Lemon Juice

1 tablespoon (1 tablespoon) Minced Garlic

2 teaspoons (2 teaspoons) Red Pepper Flakes

1 tablespoon (1 tablespoon) chopped chives, or 1 teaspoon dried chives

1 tablespoon (1 tablespoon) chopped fresh basil, or 1 teaspoon dried basil

2 tablespoons (2 tablespoons) Chicken Stock, (or white wine)

1 lb. (453.59 g) Raw Shrimp, (21-25 count)

Instructions

Turn your air fryer to 330F. Place a 6 x 3 metal pan in it and allow it to start heating while you gather your ingredients.

Place the butter, garlic, and red pepper flakes into the hot 6-inch pan.

Allow it to cook for 2 minutes, stirring once, until the butter has melted. Do not skip this step. This is what infuses garlic into the butter, which is what makes it all taste so good.

Open the air fryer, add butter, lemon juice, minced garlic, red pepper flakes, chives, basil, chicken stock, and shrimp to the pan in the order listed, stirring gently.

Allow shrimp to cook for 5 minutes, stirring once. At this point, the butter should be well-melted and liquid, bathing the shrimp in spiced goodness.

Mix very well, remove the 6-inch pan using silicone mitts, and let it rest for 1 minute on the counter. You're doing this so that you let the shrimp cook in the residual heat, rather than letting it accidentally overcook and get rubbery.

Stir at the end of the minute. The shrimp should be well-cooked at this point.

Sprinkle additional fresh basil leaves and enjoy.

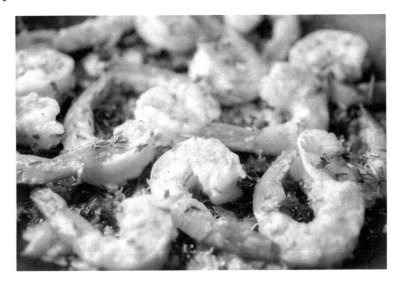

AIR FRYER CHOCOLATE COOKIES

Ingredients

½ Cup butter

⅓ Cup cream cheese

1 Egg beaten

1 Tsp vanilla extract

⅓ Cup erythritol

½ Cup coconut flour

⅓ Cup sugar-free chocolate chip cookies

Instructions

In a bowl mix butter and cream cheese. Add erythritol and vanilla extract and whip up until fluffy. Add the egg and beat until incorporated. Mix in coconut flour and chocolate chips. Let the dough rest for 10 minutes.

Scoop out around 1 Tbsp of dough and form the cookies.

Line the air fryer basket with parchment paper and place the cookies inside. Air fry for 6 minutes at 350 degrees.

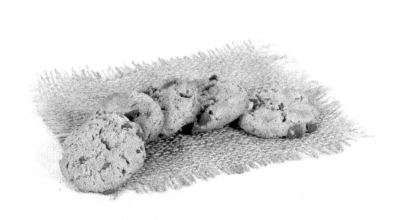

AIR FRYER SPICES CHICKEN WINGS

Prep time

10 mins

Cook time

23 mins

Marinate time

4 hrs.

Total time

4 hrs. 33 mins

Ingredients

⅓ cup extra virgin olive oil

¼ cup fresh lemon juice

2 large cloves garlic minced

2 tsp dried oregano

1 tsp fresh or ½ tsp dried thyme

2 tsp kosher salt

½ tsp coarsely ground pepper

¼ tsp crushed red pepper flakes

2 lb chicken wing drumettes

Tzatziki sauce

Instructions

Whisk together all the ingredients except the chicken and Tzaziki sauce. Put the marinade in a large resealable bag and add the chicken.

Refrigerate 4 hours to overnight, turning occasionally.

Heat air fryer to 370°F.

Add half the chicken and cook 20 minutes, turning chicken over midway.

After 20 minutes, give the air fryer basket a shake to toss the chicken a bit. Cook 2 minutes more or until juices run clear and meat is no longer pink.

Repeat with the remaining chicken. Serve with Tzatziki sauce.

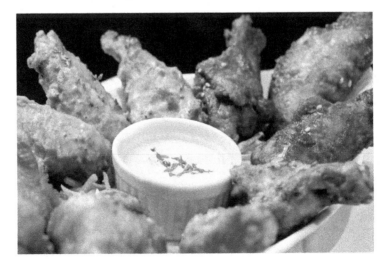

AIR FRYER LEMON ZUCCHINI

ingredients

6-7 cups zucchini (or about 6 small zucchini or 3 large zucchini), sliced into ⅛" thick coins; slice into half-coins if using large zucchini

1 tablespoon olive oil

¼ teaspoon salt

2 lemon slices (or 1.5 teaspoons lemon juice)

instructions

Preheat your air fryer to 400 degrees for 4-5 minutes.

In a medium-size mixing bowl, toss together the zucchini and olive oil until the zucchini is evenly coated in the oil. Sprinkle the salt on and toss the zucchini again until the salt is evenly distributed.

Add the zucchini to the preheated air fryer and air fry for 18-22 minutes, tossing the zucchini every 4 minutes, or until the zucchini is fried to your preferred level of doneness. I like mine super crispy and golden and usually roast for 20-22 minutes.

Squeeze the lemon juice over the zucchini, season the vegetables with extra salt if needed, and serve hot!

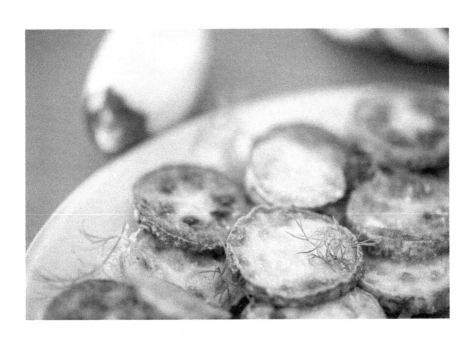

LOW CARB AIR FRYER SAUSAGE BALLS

Prep Time: 18 minutes

Cook Time: 5 minutes

Total Time: 23 minutes

Servings: 20 Piece

Ingredients

1 pound Ground Pork Sausage

1 cup Almond Flour

1 cup Shredded Cheddar Cheese

Instructions

Prepare Your Air Fryer: Grease your air fryer basket by spraying some avocado oil on the bottom. I also like using a piece of aluminum foil on the bottom in order for the oil to catch which makes for an easy clean up. You can preheat the air fryer, but it is not necessary.

Mix All Ingredients: In a medium sized bowl, add the ground sausage, cheese and almond flour and mix with your hands until all ingredients are evenly combined.

Form Sausage Balls: Form meat mixture into 1-inch balls. You could make them bigger or smaller, however make sure you adjust your

Add each sausage ball in a single layer to the basket of your air fryer and air fry at 375 degrees for 16-18 minutes or until sausage is cooked all the way through.

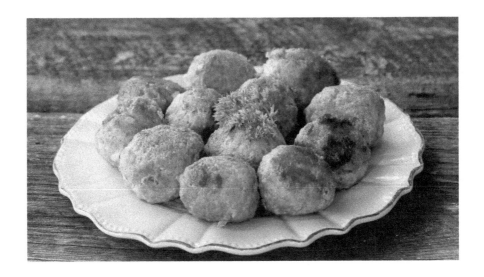

AIR FRYER ROASTED BROCCOLI

Serves: 4

Prep:10 minutes

Cook:20 minutes

TotaL:30 minutes

Ingredients

1 Lb. Broccoli, Cut into florets

1 1/2 Tbsp Peanut oil

1 Tbsp Garlic, minced

Salt

2 Tbsp Reduced sodium soy sauce

2 tsp Honey (or agave)

2 tsp Sriracha

1 tsp Rice vinegar

1/3 Cup Roasted salted peanuts

Fresh lime juice (optional)

Instructions

In a large bowl, toss together the broccoli, peanut oil, garlic and season with sea salt. Make sure the oil covers all the broccoli florets. I like to use my hands to give each one a quick rub.

Spread the broccoli into the wire basket of your air fryer, in as single of a layer, as possible, trying to leave a little bit of space between each floret.

Cook at 400 degrees until golden brown and crispy, about 15 – 20 minutes, stirring halfway.

While the broccoli cooks, mix together the honey, soy sauce, sriracha and rice vinegar in a small, microwave-safe bowl.

Once mixed, microwave the mixture for 10-15 seconds until the honey is melted, and evenly incorporated.

Transfer the cooked broccoli to a bowl and add in the soy sauce mixture. Toss to coat and season to taste with a pinch more salt, if needed.

Stir in the peanuts and squeeze lime on top (if desired.)

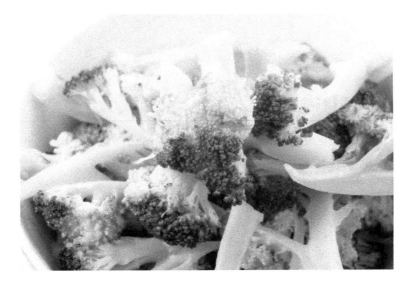

ROASTED BRUSSELS SPROUTS RECIPE

Prep Time: 10 minutes

Cook Time: 8 minutes

Total Time: 18 minutes

Servings: 4 servings

Ingredients

1 lb. brussels sprouts (cleaned and trimmed)

½ tsp. dried thyme

1 tsp. dried parsley

1 tsp. garlic powder (Or 4 cloves, minced)

¼ tsp. salt

2 tsp. oil

Instructions

Place all ingredients in a medium to large mixing bowl and toss to coat the brussels sprouts evenly.

Pour them into the food basket of the air fryer and close it up.

Set the heat to 390 F. and the time to 8 minutes. This setting roasts them nicely on the outside while leaving the insides a nicely cooked al dente.

Cool slightly and serve.

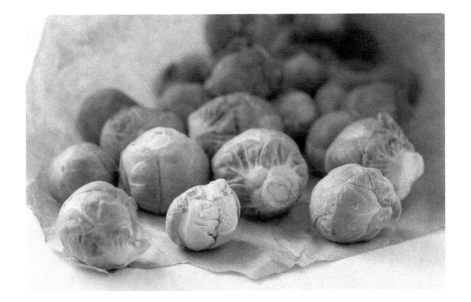

AIR FRYER CHEDDAR JALAPENO POPPERS

Prep time 10 minutes

Cook Time5 minutes

Total Time15 minutes

Servings5

Ingredients

10 fresh jalapenos

6 oz cream cheese I used reduced-fat

1/4 cup shredded cheddar cheese

2 slices bacon cooked and crumbled

cooking oil spray

Instructions

Slice the jalapenos in half, vertically, to create 2 halves per jalapeno.

Place the cream cheese in a bowl. Microwave for 15 seconds to soften.

Remove the seeds and the inside of the jalapeno. (Save some of the seeds if you prefer spicy poppers)

Combine the cream cheese, crumbled bacon, and shredded cheese in a bowl. Mix well.

For extra spicy poppers, add some of the seeds as noted above to the cream cheese mixture, and mix well.

Stuff each of the jalapenos with the cream cheese mixture.

Load the poppers into the Air Fryer. Spray the poppers with cooking oil.

Close the Air Fryer. Cook the poppers on 370 degrees for 5 minutes.

Remove from the Air Fryer and cool before serving.

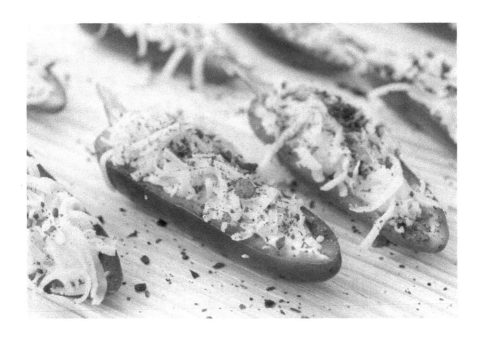

AIR FRYER BANANA BREAD

Total time: 30 minutes

Ingredients

1 el peanut oil or sunflower oil

2 ripe bananas

250 g flower

1 tl baking powder

115 g soft butter

110 g Brown sugar

100 g grated coconut

1 little hand pecans

1 Chilli (finely chopped without seeds)

2 beaten eggs

1 pinch salt

Garnish

1 ripe banana

grater of 1 orange

Instructions

Coat the XXL baking accessory with a little bit of oil.

Put all ingredients in a blender or mix the flour, baking powder and salt in a bowl. Mix the softened butter with the sugar in another bowl.

Mash the bananas with a fork (the riper the bananas, the easier this is) and mix in the beaten eggs. The finer you practice the bananas, the fewer pieces of bananas you will taste in the cake.

Add the banana-egg mixture to the sugar-butter mixture and mix well with a spatula or spoon, also add the chopped chili pepper and the coconut.

Add the flour mixture little by little, mixing again and again, then add the pecans and mix well.

Put the mixture in the XXL baking accessory and place in the Air fryer basket and bake at 160 °C for 30-35 minutes.

Check after 30 minutes if it is done by inserting a skewer; if it comes out clean, it is ready. Otherwise, put an extra 5 minutes in the Air fryer.

When the banana bread has cooled, cut a slice and grate your orange zest over it.

Enjoy!

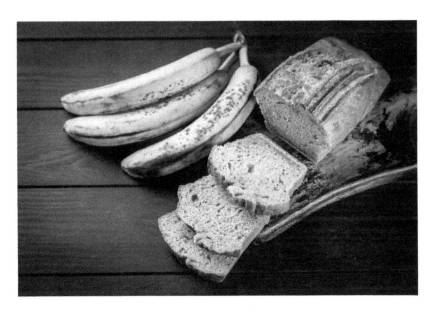

AIR FRYER TEXAS TOAST STICKS

Cooking Time: 5 Min

Servings: 15

Ingredients

• Four pieces of slightly stale thick bread, like Texas toast

• Parchment paper

• Two eggs, lightly crushed

• 1/4 cup milk

 (optional)   • 1 tsp. vanilla extract

• 1 tsp. cinnamon

• One pinch of ground nutmeg

Instructions

First slice each piece of bread into thirds to create sticks. Cut a sheet of parchment paper to fit the base of the air fryer basket.

Preheat air fryer to 360 degrees F (180 degrees C).

Mix together eggs, vanilla, vanilla extract, cinnamon, and nutmeg in a bowl till well blended. Into the egg mixture, dip each slice of bread, ensuring every piece is nicely submerged. Shake every breadstick to get rid of excess liquid and set it in one layer in the air fryer basket. Cook in batches, if necessary, to prevent overcrowding the fryer.

Then cook for 5 minutes, then turn bread bits and cook for another five minutes.

BAKED EGG AND HAM CUP

Cooking Time: 10 min

Servings: 2

Ingredients:

- 1 egg

- 1 cup ham, chopped

- ½ onion, chopped

- 1 tbsp. butter

- 1/3 cup parmesan, grated

Instructions

Start by preheating your fryer to 350°F.

Then whisk the egg into a bowl well before adding in the ham, onion, and butter. Combine well and add seasoning if desired.

Scoop equal portions into three ramekins, adding a sprinkle of parmesan on top.

Then place into the fryer and cook for ten minutes. Take care when removing the ramekins, and serve hot.

AIR FRIED TASTY CHICKEN DRUMSTICKS

Prep time: 5 minutes

Cook time: 25 minutes

Total time: 30 minutes

Ingredients

8 chicken drumsticks

2 tbsp olive oil

1 tsp celtic sea salt

1 tsp fresh cracked pepper

1 tsp garlic powder

1 tsp paprika

1/2 tsp cumin

Instructions

In a small bowl, combine herbs and spices.

Set aside.

Place drumsticks in a bowl or a plastic bag and drizzle with olive oil.

Toss to coat.

Sprinkle herbs and spices all over drumsticks to coat them.

Preheat air fryer at 400 for 2-10 minutes.

Place drumsticks in air fryer basket and cook for 10 minutes on 400.

Remove basket and flip chicken drumsticks.

Cook at 400 for another 10 minutes.

If chicken is not 165 degrees internally, add another 5 minutes of cook-time.

Time can vary based on drumstick size, so do check the temperature with a digital thermometer after cooking to prevent over or under cooking.

When chicken has reached 165 degrees internally, serve immediately.

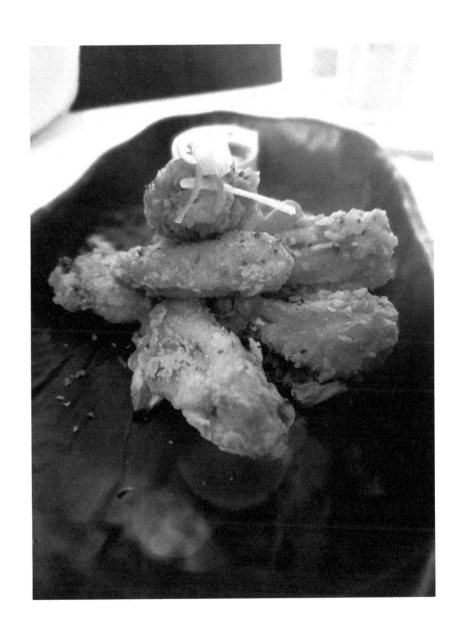

MINCED GARLIC MEATBALLS

Cooking time: 20 min Servings: 4

Ingredients:

½ -pound. boneless chicken thighs

1 tsp. minced garlic

one ¼ cup roasted pecans

½ cup mushrooms

1 tsp. extra virgin olive oil

Instruction

start by preheating your fryer to 375°f.

cube the chicken thighs.

then position them in the food processor along with the garlic, pecans, and other seasonings as desired. pulse until a smooth consistency is achieved.

chop the mushrooms finely. add to the chicken mixture and combine.

with the use of your hands, shape the mixture into balls and brush them with olive oil.

and put the balls into the fryer and cook for eighteen minutes. serve hot.

CRISPY SOUTHERN FRIED CHICKEN

Cooking Time: 25 min

Servings: 6

Ingredients

2 x 6-oz. boneless skinless chicken breasts

2 tbsp. hot sauce

½ tsp. onion powder

1 tbsp. chili powder

2 oz. pork rinds, finely ground

Instruction

Start Slicing the chicken breasts in ½ lengthwise and rub in the hot sauce. Then combine the onion powder with the chili powder, and then rub it into the chicken. Let it marinate for at least a half-hour.

After that use the ground pork rinds to coat the chicken breasts in the ground pork rinds, covering them thoroughly. Place the chicken in your fryer.

Set the fryer at 350°F and cook the chicken for 13 minutes. Turnover the chicken and cook the other side for another 13 minutes or until golden.

Test the chicken with a meat thermometer and when it is fully cooked, it should reach 165°F. Serve hot with the sides of your choice.

ROASTED BRUSSELS SPROUTS

Preparation Time: 8 minutes Cooking Time: 20 minutes Servings: 4

Ingredients:

1 pound fresh Brussels sprouts

1 tbsp. olive oil

½ tsp. salt

1/8 tsp. pepper

¼ cup grated Parmesan cheese

Instructions

Cut the bottoms from the Brussels sprouts and pull off any discolored leaves. Toss with the olive oil, salt, and pepper, and place in the air fryer basket.

Roast for 20 minutes, shaking the air fryer basket twice during the cooking time until the Brussels sprouts are dark golden brown and crisp.

Move the Brussels sprouts to a serving dish and toss with the Parmesan cheese. Serve immediately.

Did You Know? Brussels sprouts were cultivated in Roman times and introduced into the United States in the 1880s. Most Brussels sprouts in this country are grown in California.

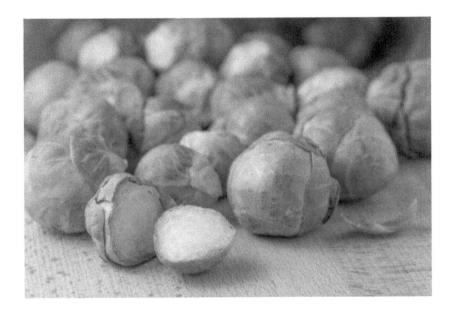

RASPBERRY-EGG FRENCH TOAST

Cooking Time: 8 min

Servings: 4

Ingredients:

•4 (1-inch-thick) slices French bread

•2 tbsps. raspberry jam

•1/3 cup fresh raspberries

•Two egg yolks

•1/3 cup 2% milk

•1 tbsp. sugar

•½ tsp. vanilla extract

•3 tbsps. sour cream

Instructions

First on either side of each bread slice, cut a pocket, making sure you don't cut through to the other side.

And in a small bowl, combine the raspberry jam and raspberries and crush the raspberries into the jam with a fork.

Then add in a shallow bowl, beat the egg yolks with the milk, sugar, and vanilla until combined.

Spread some of the sour creams in the pocket you cut in the bread slices, and then add the raspberry mixture. Squeeze the edges of the bread slightly to close the opening.

And the dip the bread in the egg mixture, letting the bread stand in the egg for 3 minutes. Flip the bread over and let it stand on the other side for 3 minutes.

Set or preheat the air fryer to 375°F. Arrange the stuffed bread in the air fryer basket in a single layer.

Air fry for 5 minutes, then carefully flip the bread slices and cook for another 3 to 6 minutes, until the French toast is golden brown.

TASTY PEPPER EGG BITES

Cooking Time: 15 min

Servings: 7

Ingredients:

•Five large eggs, beaten

•3 tbsps. 2% milk

•½ tsp. dried marjoram

•1/8 tsp. salt

•Pinch freshly ground black pepper

•1/3 cup minced bell pepper, any color

•3 tbsps. minced scallions

•½ cup shredded Colby or Muenster cheese

Instructions

Then combine the eggs, milk, marjoram, salt, and black pepper in a medium bowl, mix until combined.

Stir in the bell peppers, scallions, and cheese. Fill the seven egg bite cups with the egg mixture, making sure you get some of the solids in each cup. Set or preheat the air fryer to 325°F.

Make a foil sling: Fold an 18-inch-long piece of heavy-duty aluminum foil lengthwise into thirds. Put the egg bite pan on this sling and lower it into the air fryer.

After that leave the foil in the air fryer, but bend down the edges to fit in the appliance.

Bake the egg bites for 10 to 15 minutes or until a toothpick inserted into the center comes out clean.

Use the foil sling to remove the egg bite pan. Let cool for 5 minutes, and then invert the pan onto a plate to remove the egg bites. Serve warm.

SUMMER SQUASH FRITTATA

Cooking Time:25 min

Servings: 4

Ingredients

•¼ cup chopped red bell pepper

•¼ cup chopped yellow summer squash

•2 tbsps. chopped scallion

•2 tbsps. butter

•Five large eggs, beaten

•¼ tsp. sea salt

•1/8 tsp. freshly ground black pepper

•1 cup shredded Cheddar cheese, divided

Instructions

In a 7-inch cake pan, combine the bell pepper, summer squash, and scallion. Add the butter.

Start by preheating the air fryer to 350°F. Set the cake pan in the air fryer basket. Cook the vegetables for 3 to 4 minutes or until they are crisp- tender. Remove the pan from the air fryer.

And use salt and pepper, beat the eggs in a medium bowl. Stir in half of the Cheddar. Pour into the pan with the vegetables.

Then return the pan to the air fryer, cook for 10 to 15 minutes, and then top the frittata with the remaining cheese. Cook for another 4 to 5 minutes or until the cheese is melted and the frittata is set. Cut into wedges to serve.

PAPRIKA CHICKEN LEGS

Prep Time

10 mins

Cook Time

20 mins

Total Time

30 mins

Servings: 4 Calories: 245kcal

Ingredients

6-8 chicken drumsticks

2 tablespoons olive oil

1/2 teaspoon paprika

1/2 teaspoon garlic powder

1/2 teaspoon salt

1/4 teaspoon ground black pepper

Instructions

Preheat air fryer for 2-5 minutes.

Pat drumsticks dry with paper towel. In a small bowl, mix paprika, garlic powder, salt and pepper.

Place chicken in a large bowl or food storage bag. Pour oil and spices over chicken. Mix around until chicken is coated.

Add chicken to air fryer basket. Cook at 390 degrees for 10 minutes. Flip drumsticks over and cook for another 10 minutes at 390 degrees F.

Serve warm.

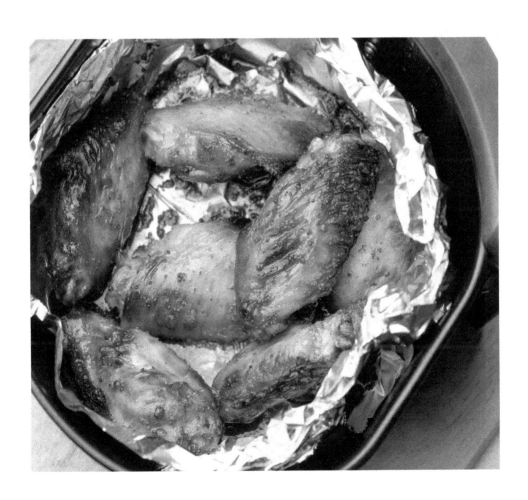

DELICIOUS PAPRIKA VEGETABLES

Cooking Time: 45 min

Servings:2

Ingredients:

Two garlic cloves, chopped

Three russet potatoes

2 oz. onions, chopped

1/4 cup red peppers, chopped

2 tsp. olive oil

1/4 tsp. salt

2 oz. cup green peppers, chopped

1 tsp. paprika seasoning

6 cups cold water

1/8 tsp. pepper

Instructions

First Scrub the potatoes and remove the skins with a knife or vegetable peeler.

Use a cheese grater to shred the potatoes completely with the largest holes available. Transfer the potatoes to a glass dish.

Then empty the cold water into the dish and saturate for approximately 20 minutes.

Empty the potatoes and remove the moisture thoroughly.

Set the temperature of the air to heat at 400°F.

In an additional glass dish, add potatoes, olive oil, salt, garlic powder, paprika powder, and pepper until completely covered.

Place the potatoes in the air fryer basket and steam for 10 minutes.

Open the lid and combine the onion, garlic, and peppers to the basket. Toss ingredients to incorporate.

Then heat for an additional 10 minutes and take out of the basket.

Wait for approximately 5 minutes before serving.

HEALTHY AIR FRYER CHICKEN FAJITAS

Prep Time: 5 minutes Cook Time: 15 minutes Total Time: 20 minutes

Servings: 8

Ingredients

2 chicken breasts boneless and skinless, cut into strips (around 1 pound/450g)

1 red bell pepper sliced into ½ inch slices

yellow bell pepper sliced into ½ inch slices

1 green bell pepper sliced into ½ inch slices

1 red onion sliced into wedges

3 tablespoons fajita seasoning

1 tablespoon vegetable oil

Instructions

Preheat the Air Fryer to 390°F (200°C).

Drizzle oil over the chicken strips, and season with the fajita seasoning. Toss well and make sure that they're evenly coated with the seasoning. Add the veggies, and season well. Make sure that everything is well coated in fajita seasoning.

Put everything in an Air Fryer basket. Air Fry at for 15 minutes, tossing halfway through.

Serve with warmed tortillas, pico de gallo, avocado slices or guacamole.

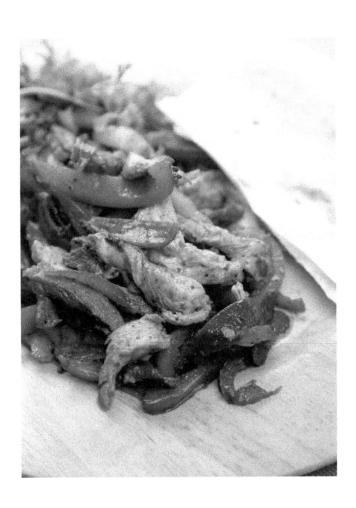

AIR FRYER PASTA WITH CHEESE

Prep Time: 10 minutes
Cook Time: 45 minutes

Ingredients

½ pound dry uncooked pasta (we used elbow macaroni)

2 cups whole milk

1 cup chicken stock

4 tablespoons butter

4 tablespoons cream cheese

8-ounce package sharp cheddar cheese, shredded

1 cup shredded mozzarella cheese

¼ teaspoon kosher salt

¼ teaspoon white pepper

1 teaspoon dry mustard

Pinch Cayenne pepper

Few grinds fresh nutmeg

Instructions

Preheat air fryer on 400 degrees F. for 10 minutes.

Rinse pasta under hot tap water for two minutes and drain.

Place milk, chicken stock, butter and cream cheese in a glass 4-cup or larger measuring cup and microwave until hot, and the butter melted, about 3-4 minutes. (This just needs to be hot enough to melt the butter and cream cheese, not boiling hot)

Mix drained pasta, hot liquid, cheddar, mozzarella, salt, pepper, mustard, cayenne and nutmeg in a large bowl then pour into the Air Fryer handled pan.

Spray a round parchment circle with pan spray and place sprayed side down over the macaroni mixture, pressing down to touch the mixture. Cover the top with foil and set into the heated air fryer and cook for 45 minutes.

Note: Air fryer wattages vary so check at 35 minutes and cook the additional 5-10 minutes as needed. Our air fryer is an 1800-watt air fryer and our macaroni and cheese took exactly 45 minutes.

Remove foil and parchment, stir and serve.

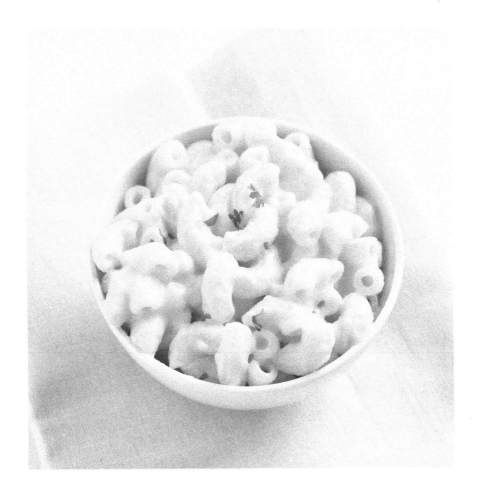

THE ESSENTIAL AIR FRYER COOKBOOK 2021

Delicious Recipes for Quick and Easy Meals. What and How to Prepare for the Best Results with Lots of Low Carb Recipes that Will Help You Stay Healthy and Lose Weight.

Violet H.Scott

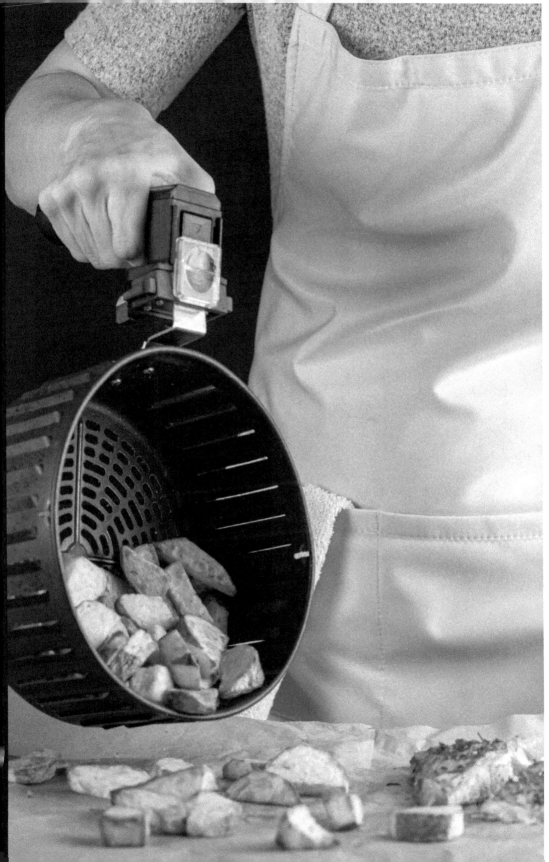

Introduction

Air fryer, what is it?

The air fryer is basically an upgraded tabletop ventilation oven. This small device aims to achieve frying results with only hot air and very little or no oil.

This device has become very popular in recent years - about 45% of US homes have one. There are all kinds of things you can air-fry, from frozen chicken wings to French fries, from roasted vegetables to freshly baked cookies.

It allows you to cook food within a stream of hot air. In this process, the food is spun in this stream of air and then fried. Compared to traditional fryers, there is no need for much fat. Today's technology allows for the preparation of delicacies that retain their natural taste.

Recipes

AIR FRYER MUSHROOMS

Yield: 2 servings

 Prep time: 10 mins Cook time: 15 mins Total time: 25 mins

Ingredients

8 oz. (227 g) mushrooms, washed and dried

1-2 Tablespoons (15-30 ml) olive oil

1/2 teaspoon (2.5 ml) garlic powder

1 teaspoon (5 ml) Worcestershire or soy sauce

Kosher salt, to taste

black pepper, to taste

lemon wedges (optional)

1 Tablespoon (15 ml) chopped parsley

Instructions

Make sure mushrooms are evenly cut for even cooking. Cut mushrooms in half or quarters (depending on preferred size). Add to bowl then toss with oil, garlic powder, Worcestershire/soy sauce, salt and pepper

Air fry at 380°F for 10-12 minutes, tossing and shaking half way through. Adjust cooking time to your preferred doneness.

Drizzle and squeeze some fresh lemon juice and top with chopped parsley. Serve warm. Yum!

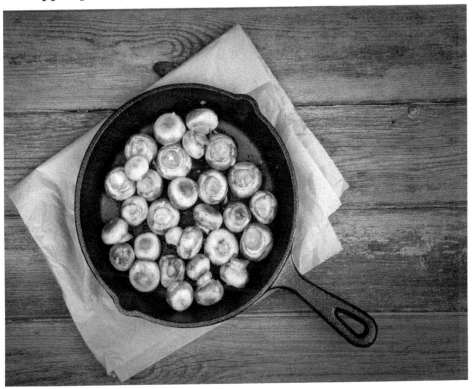

WHOLE GRILLED CHICKEN

Servings 3-4,

Preparation: 5 min

 Cooking time 30-40 min

Ingredients

1 whole chicken (about 800 g)

2 tablespoons olive oil

Salt

Pepper

Fresh thyme

1 whole garlic

1 lemon

Instructions

Rinse the chicken in cold water and pat it dry with kitchen paper.

2. Then brush or rub the oil over the whole chicken.

3. Salt and pepper

4. Place the thyme sprigs in the bottom of the Air fryer basket, and place the chicken on top.

5. Divide the lemon in half and rub the juice of one half over the chicken, and place the other half in the basket next to the chicken.

Divide the garlic in half and place them in the basket together with the chicken.

Cook in the Air fryer at 180 ° C, 30-40 minutes.

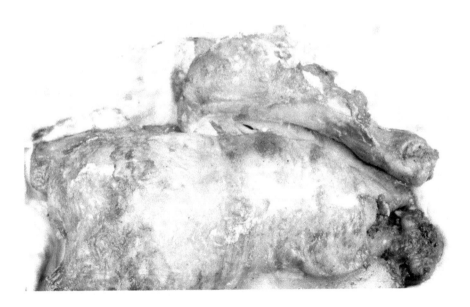

AIR FRYER LIGHT ASPARAGUS

Prep Time: 4 minutes Cook Time: 7 minutes

Servings: 4 Calories: 55kcal

Ingredients

1 lb asparagus

1/4 tsp salt

1/8 tsp black pepper

1 Tbsp avocado oil

1 garlic clove pressed

Instructions

Start by snapping off the end of each asparagus spare. The ends tend to be quite chewy so you want to get rid of them. You want to remove about 1 to 2 inches from the bottom.

Now place the trimmed asparagus on a rimmed baking sheet and drizzle with avocado oil. Then mix in the pressed or grated garlic clove.

Now season with salt and pepper and toss them until they are well coated in the seasoning.

Place the seasoned asparagus on the air fryer basket and cook on high (450 degrees) for 7 minutes.

Enjoy!

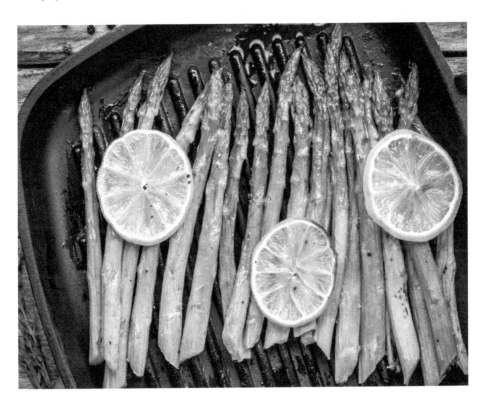

KETO ZUCCHINI FRIES

yield: 6 SERVINGS prep time: 15 MINUTES cook time: 25 MINUTES total time: 40 MINUTE

Ingredients

2 medium zucchini

1 egg

1/4 tsp salt

1 cup almond flour

1/2 cup grated Parmesan cheese

1 tsp garlic powder

1 tsp Italian herb blend

Instructions

Preheat the oven to 425 degrees Fahrenheit and line a large baking sheet with parchment paper.

Slice the zucchini in half crosswise. Then, cut again lengthwise into sticks.

Crack the egg in a shallow bowl and lightly beat it with the salt.

Add the almond flour, parmesan, garlic, and herbs to a separate shallow bowl and stir to combine.

Using one hand, dip a piece of zucchini in the egg wash, let excess egg drip off, and transfer to the almond/parmesan mixture. Using your other hand, press the zucchini in the almond/parmesan mixture to coat. Place on the baking sheet in a single layer. Repeat this process until all zucchini pieces are coated. Spray with olive oil.

Bake for 25-30 minutes, flipping halfway through. Serve immediately.

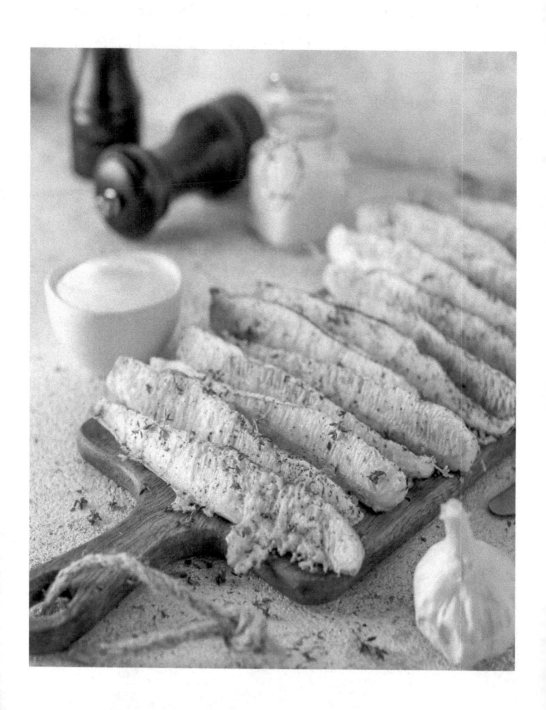

YUMMY SLICED BACON

Cooking Time: 10 min

Servings: 2

Ingredients

•Brown sugar - 3 tbsp.

•Water - 2 tbsp.

•Eight slices bacon

•Maple syrup - 2 tbsp.

Instructions

First adjust the air fryer to heat at 400°F. Remove the basket and cover the base with baking paper.

Then empty the water into the base of the fryer while preheating.

In a glass dish add and whisk the 2 tbsp. Of maple syrup and the 3 tbsp. Brown sugar together.

Place the wire rack into the basket and arrange the bacon into a single layer.

After that spread the sugar glaze on the bacon until completely covered.

Then put the basket into the air fryer and steam for 8 minutes.

Then move the bacon from the basket and wait about 5 minutes before serving hot.

AIR FRYER POTATOES CHIPS

Prep Time

15 mins

Cook Time

25 mins

Total Time

40 mins

Ingredients

4 medium yellow potatoes

1 tbsp oil

salt to taste

Instructions

Slice the potatoes into thin slices. Place them into a bowl with cold water and let it soak for at least 20 minutes.

Remove from water, pat dry with a towel.

Season the potato chips with salt and oil. Place them in an air fryer and cook for 20 minutes at 200°F.

Toss the potato chips, turn up heat to 400°F and cook for about 5 more minutes

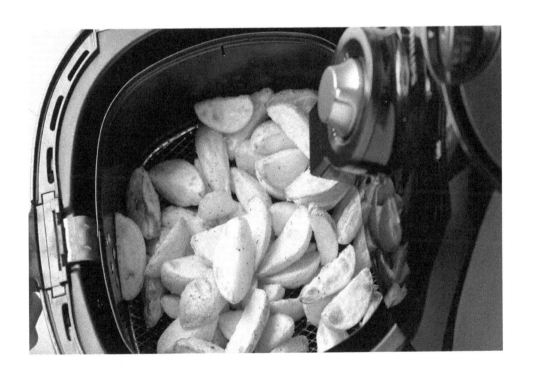

AIR FRYER ONION RINGS

Prep Time

20 mins

Cook Time

10 mins

Total Time

30 mins

Servings: 6

Ingredients

1 large sweet onion cut into rings

1 cup almond flour

1 cup grated Parmesan cheese

1 tablespoon baking powder

1 teaspoon smoked paprika

Salt and pepper

2 eggs beaten

1 tablespoon heavy cream

cooking spray

Instructions

In a medium bowl, combine the almond flour, Parmesan cheese, baking powder, smoked paprika, salt, and pepper.

Beat the eggs and heavy cream in another bowl.

Dip the onion rings in the eggs and then in the almond flour mixture. Press the almond flour mixture into the onions. Transfer to a parchment lined baking sheet and repeat with the remaining onion.

Air Fryer Instructions

Preheat your air fryer to 350 degrees. Arrange the onions in a single layer, cooking in batches as needed. (If desired, you can line your air fryer with air fryer liners.)

Spray the onions with cooking spray and cook for 5 minutes. Use a spatula to carefully reach under the onions and flip. Respray and cook 5 minutes longer.

Baking Instructions

Preheat the oven to 400 degrees. Line a baking sheet with parchment paper. Arrange the onions in a single layer and spray with cooking spray. Bake for 10 minutes. Flip and respray with oil. Bake another 10 to 12 minutes, until crispy and brown.

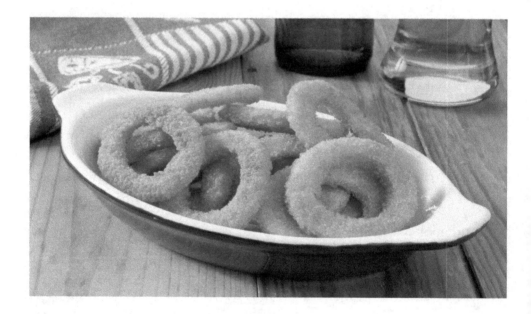

YUMMY BACON-WRAPPED DATES

Cooking Time: 6 min Servings: 6

Ingredients:

•12 dates, pitted

•Six slices of high-quality bacon, cut in half

•Cooking spray

Instructions

Start by preheating the air fryer oven to 360°F (182°C).

Then use half a bacon slice to wrap each date and secure it with a toothpick.

Spritz the air fryer basket using cooking spray, and then place bacon- wrapped dates in the basket.

Put the air fryer basket and the select Air Fry, and set the time to 6 minutes, or until the bacon is crispy.

Remove the dates and allow cooling on a wire rack for 5 minutes before serving.

TASTY BACON-WRAPPED SHRIMP

Cooking Time: 13 min Servings: 8

Ingredients:

- 24 large shrimp, peeled and deveined, about ¾ pound (340 g)
- Five tbsps. barbecue sauce, divided
- 12 strips bacon, cut in half
- 24 small pickled jalapeño slices

Instructions

First you need to toss together the shrimp and 3 tbsps. Of the barbecue sauce. Let stand for 15 minutes. Soak 24 wooden toothpicks in water for 10 minutes. Wrap one piece of bacon around the shrimp and jalapeño slice, then secure with a toothpick.

Start by preheating the air fryer oven, set the temperature to 350°F (177°C).

Then place the shrimp in the air fryer basket, spacing them ½ inch apart, select Air Fry, and set time to 10 minutes.

Turn shrimp over with tongs and air fry for 3 minutes more, or until bacon is golden brown and shrimp are cooked through.

Brush with the remaining barbecue sauce and serve.

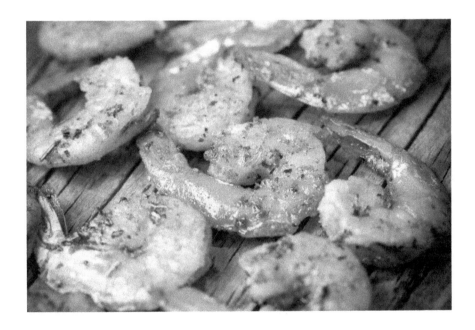

AIR FRYER CHILI SHRIMP

Prep Time

10 mins

Cook Time

12 mins

0 mins

Total Time

22 mins

Servings: 4 servings

Ingredients

1 pound shrimp raw, large, peeled and deveined with tails attached

¼ cup all-purpose flour

½ teaspoon salt

¼ teaspoon black pepper

2 large eggs

¾ cup unsweetened shredded coconut

¼ cup panko breadcrumbs

Cooking spray

Sweet chili sauce for serving

Instructions

Preheat the air fryer to 360°F. When heated, spray the basket with cooking spray.

Combine the flour, salt and pepper in one shallow bowl. Whisk the eggs in a second shallow bowl. Then combine the shredded coconut and panko breadcrumbs in a third shallow bowl.

Dip the shrimp into the flour mixture, shaking off any excess. Then dredge the shrimp into the eggs, and finally into the coconut panko mixture, gently pressing to adhere.

Place the coconut shrimp in the air fryer so they are not touching, and spray the top of the shrimp. Cook for 10-12 minutes, flipping halfway through.

Garnish with chopped parsley, and serve immediately with sweet chili sauce, if desired.

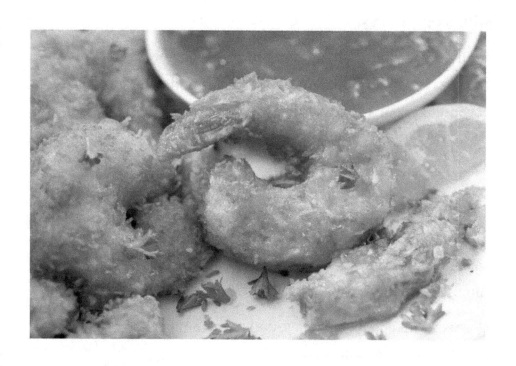

TASTY SWEET POTATO TOAST

Cooking Time:30 Min   Servings:2

Ingredients

- Salt - 1/4 tsp.
- Paprika seasoning - 1/8 tsp.
- Avocado oil - 4 tsp.
- Garlic powder - 1/8 tsp.
- Onion powder - 1/8 tsp.
- Pepper - 1/4 tsp.
- Oregano seasoning - 1/8 tsp.

- One sweet potato

Instructions

Start by heating the air fryer to the temperature of 380°F.

Then cut the ends off the sweet potato and discard. Divide into four even pieces lengthwise.

And whisk the avocado oil and all of the seasonings until combined thoroughly.

Brush the spices on top of the slices of sweet potato.

After that transfer the slices to the air fryer basket and fry for 15 minutes.

Turn the sweet potato pieces over and steam once again for 15 more minutes.

Remove to a serving plate and enhance with your preferred toppings.

AIR FRYER KALE CHIPS

prep time: 5 MINUTES cook time: 7 MINUTES total time: 12 MINUTES

ingredients

1 batch curly kale, washed and patted dry

2 teaspoons olive oil

1 tablespoon nutritional yeast

¼ teaspoon sea salt

1/8 teaspoon ground black pepper

instructions

Remove the leaves from the stems of the kale and place them in a medium bowl.

Add the olive oil, nutritional yeast, salt, and pepper. Use your hands to massage the toppings into the kale leaves.

Pour the kale into the basket of your air fryer and cook on 390 degrees F for 6-7 minutes, or until they are crispy.

Serve warm or at room temperature.

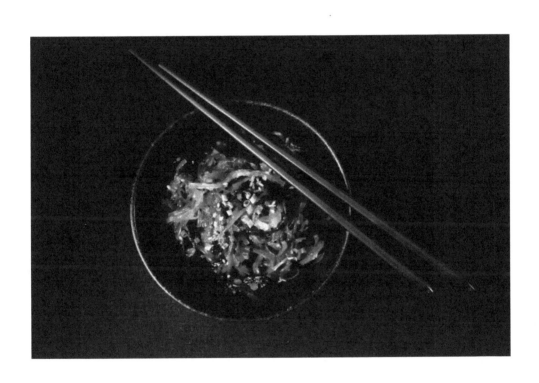

ROASTED BELL PEPPERS

Preparation Time: 8 minutes Cooking Time: 22 minutes
Servings: 4

Ingredients:

One red bell pepper

One yellow bell pepper

One orange bell pepper

One green bell pepper

2 tbsps. olive oil, divided

½ tsp. dried marjoram

Pinch salt

Freshly ground black pepper

One head garlic

Instructions

Slice the bell peppers into 1-inch strips.

In a prepared large bowl, toss the bell peppers with 1 tbsp of the oil. Sprinkle on the marjoram, salt, and pepper, and toss again.

Trim the top of the head of the garlic and place the cloves on an oiled square of aluminum foil. Drizzle with the remaining olive oil. Wrap the garlic in the foil.

Place the wrapped garlic in the air fryer and roast for 15 minutes, then add the bell peppers. Roast for 7 minutes or until the peppers are tender and the garlic is soft. Transfer the peppers to a serving dish.

Remove the garlic from the air fryer and unwrap the foil. When cool enough to handle, squeeze the garlic cloves out of the papery skin and mix with the bell peppers.

Cooking tip: To easily remove the seeds from a dash of bell pepper, cut around the stem with a sharp knife and simply pull out the stem with the seeds attached. Rinse the pepper to remove any stray seeds and cut them into strips.

AIR-FRIED BROCCOLI CRISPS

Preparation Time: 10 minutes

Cooking Time: 12 minutes

Servings: 4

Ingredients

One large broccoli head, chopped

2 tbsps. olive oil

1 tsp. black pepper

1 tsp. salt

Instructions:

Set your Air Fryer Oven temperature to 360 degrees F

Take a bowl and add broccoli florets, olive oil, salt, and black pepper

Then toss them well

Add the broccoli florets

Cook for 12 minutes

Shake after 6 minutes

Remove it from your air fryer and let it cool before serve

Serve and enjoy!

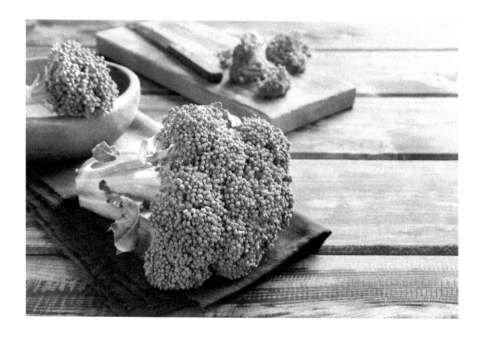

CRISPY KETO CROUTONS

Prep time10 minutes Cook time10 minutes Total time 20 minutes

Ingredients

2 Cups of Keto Farmers Bread (200g) half of the loaf

1 Tbsp of Marjoram

2Tbsp Olive Oil

1/2 Tbsp Garlic Powder

Instructions

As I have already mentioned our Keto Farmers Bread is used in this recipe.

Make sure your bread is cooled. Cut it into same size slices and then squares.

Place all of the croutons into a big bowl, which would be spacious enough to mix all the herbs and oil.

Add oil, Dry Garlic and Marjoram.

With a big spatula, mix all of the croutons fully. Do not forget to make sure the oil and herbs are spread evenly.

Depending on your Air Fryer, fill it up with your Keto Croutons. Make sure you only add one layer, otherwise they will not crisp fully.

Switch the Air Fryer on. You do not need to add additional oil, since you have already coated your Keto Croutons with oil before.

After 10 minutes the Crunchy Keto Croutons are ready to be served. Let them cool or serve them still hot or warm. It all depends for what you want to use them.

Bon Appetit

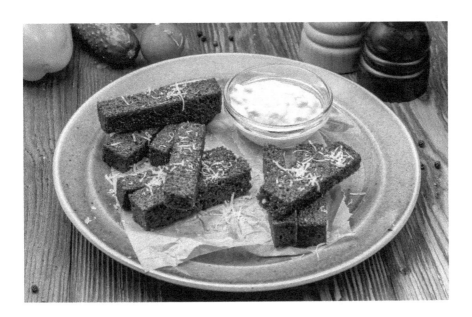

TASTY APPLE CHEESE

Cooking Time: 5 min Servings: 8 roll-ups

Ingredients:

Eight slices whole wheat sandwich bread

4 ounces (113 g) Colby Jack cheese, grated

½ small apple, chopped

2 tbsps. butter, melted

Instructions

Start by preheating the air fryer oven to 390°F (199°C).

Take the crusts from the bread and flatten the slices with a rolling pin. Don't be gentle. Press hard so that the bread will be very thin.

Then top the bread slices with cheese and chopped apple, dividing the ingredients evenly.

After that roll up each slice tightly and secure each with one or two toothpicks.

Brush outside of rolls with melted butter. Place them in the air fryer basket.

Putting the air fryer basket onto the baking pan and select Air Fry, and set time to 5 minutes, or until outside is crisp and nicely browned.

Serve hot.

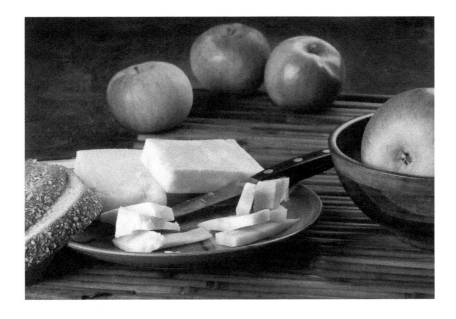

YUMMY AND CHEESY HASH BROWN BRUSCHETTA

Cooking Time: 8 min Servings: 4

Ingredients:

Four frozen hash brown patties

1 tbsp. olive oil

1/3 cup chopped cherry tomatoes

3 tbsps. diced fresh Mozzarella

2 tbsps. grated Parmesan cheese

1 tbsp. balsamic vinegar

1 tbsp. minced fresh basil

Instructions

Start by preheating the air fryer oven temperature to 400°F (204°C).

Put the hash brown patties in the air fryer basket in a single layer.

Then put the air fryer basket onto the baking pan and select Air Fry, set time to 8 minutes, or wait until the potatoes are crisp, hot, and golden brown.

In the meantime and combine the olive oil, tomatoes, Mozzarella, Parmesan, vinegar, and basil in a small bowl.

When the potatoes are finished, you can remove them from the basket carefully and arrange them on a serving plate. Top with the tomato mixture and serve.

PAPRIKA PORK CHOPS

Prep Time 5 minutes

Cook Time 12 minutes

Servings 4

Ingredients

8 oz pork chops (four) bone-in center-cut, or boneless (see recipe notes)

1 tsp olive oil

Pork Chop Seasoning

1 tsp paprika

1 tsp onion powder

1 tsp salt

1 tsp pepper

instructions

Preheat your air fryer to 380°F.

Brush both sides of pork chop with a little olive oil.

Mix the pork seasonings together in a bowl (this is enough for four pork chops) and apply to both sides of the pork chop.

Place pork chop in air fryer and cook for between 9-12 minutes, turning the chop over halfway, until it reaches a minimum temp of 145°F (exact cook time will vary depending on thickness of pork and your model of air fryer)

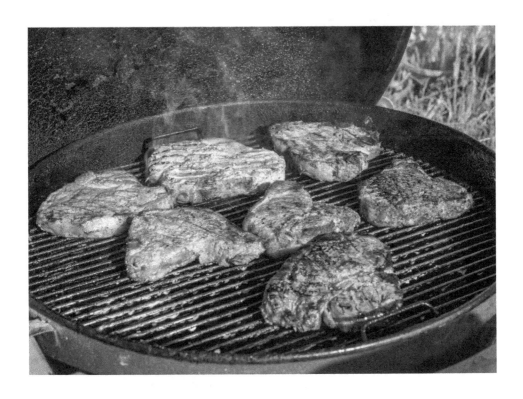

EGGPLANT SIDE DISH

Preparation Time: 10 minutes Cooking Time: 10 minutes
Servings: 4

Ingredients

Eight baby eggplants

½ tsp. garlic powder

One yellow onion, chopped

One green bell pepper, chopped

One bunch coriander, chopped

1 tbsp. tomato paste

1 tbsp. olive oil

One tomato, chopped

Salt and black pepper

Instructions

Place a pan over heat and then add the oil.

Melt the oil and fry the onion for 1 minute

Add green bell pepper, oregano, eggplant pulp, tomato, coriander, garlic powder, tomato paste, salt, and pepper. Stir-fry for 2 minutes

Remove from the heat and let it cool

Arrange them in your Air fryer

Cook for 8 minutes at 360 degrees F

Serve and enjoy!

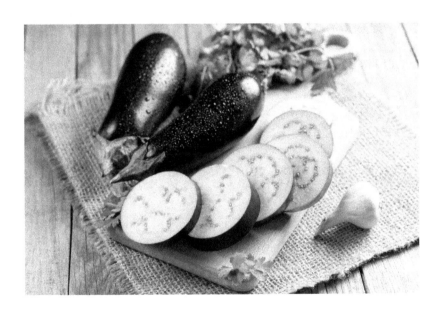

SANDWICHES NUTS & CHEESE

Preparation Time: 10 minutes Cooking Time: 50 minutes
Servings: 2

Ingredients

One heirloom tomato

1 (4-oz) block feta cheese

One small red onion, thinly sliced

One clove garlic

Salt to taste

2 tsp. + ¼ cup olive oil

1 ½ tbsp. toasted pine nuts

¼ cup chopped parsley

¼ cup grated Parmesan cheese

¼ cup chopped basil

Instructions

Add basil, pine nuts, garlic, and salt to a food processor. Process while slowly adding ¼ cup of olive oil. Once finished, pour basil pesto into a bowl and refrigerate for 30 minutes.

Preheat on Air Fry function to 390 F. Slice the feta cheese and tomato into ½-inch slices. Remove the pesto from the fridge and spread half of it on the tomato slices. Top with feta cheese slices and onion. Drizzle the remaining olive oil on top.

Place the tomatoes in the fryer basket and fit in the baking tray; cook for 12 minutes. Remove to a serving platter and top with the remaining pesto. Serve.

AIR FRYER BROCCOLI

Prep time 5 minutes

Cook time 6 minutes

Total time 11 minutes

Yield: 4 servings

Ingredients

1 head of broccoli

2 tablespoons butter, melted

1 clove garlic, minced

salt and pepper to taste

1/4 cup Parmesan cheese (freshly grated)

additional parmesan cheese for serving

pinch of red pepper flakes (optional)

Instructions

Preheat your air fryer to 400 degrees.

Cut broccoli into florets and set aside.

Mix together melted butter, minced garlic, salt, pepper, and red pepper flakes (if using).

Add the broccoli and mix to combine thoroughly.

Add the Parmesan cheese and mix again making sure to coat it evenly.

Place broccoli into the air fryer and cook for 6-8 minutes, shaking the basket halfway through. *

Remove broccoli from the air fryer and serve immediately.

Add additional Parmesan cheese on top once served.

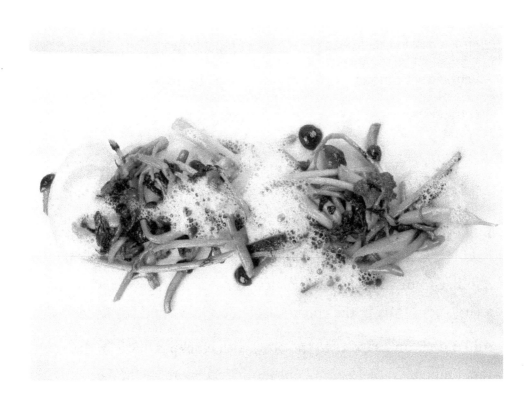

CHICKPEA & CARROT BALLS

Preparation Time: 5 minutes Cooking Time: 20 minutes
Servings: 3

Ingredients

2 tbsp. olive oil

2 tbsp. soy sauce

1 tbsp. flax meal

2 cups cooked chickpeas

½ cup sweet onions

½ cup grated carrots

½ cup roasted cashews

Juice of 1 lemon

½ tsp. turmeric

1 tsp. cumin

1 tsp. garlic powder

1 cup rolled oats

Instructions

Combine the olive oil, onions, and carrots into the Air Fryer baking pan and cook them on Air Fry function for 6 minutes at 350 F. Ground the oats and cashews in a food processor. Place in a large bowl. Mix in the chickpeas, lemon juice, and soy sauce.

Add onions and carrots to the bowl with chickpeas. Stir in the remaining ingredients; mix until fully incorporated. Make meatballs out of the mixture. Increase the temperature to 370 F and cook for 12 minutes

SUCCULENT CHICKEN NUGGETS FOR AIR FRYER

Prep time 5 mins Cook Time 10 mins Yields 4 servings

Ingredients

1 lb. chicken tenders

1 tbsp chicken seasoning

1 tbsp olive oil

Instructions

Preheat air fryer to 400°F/200°C. If your air fryer doesn't have this function, let it run empty for 5 minutes.

Add your chicken tenders to a bowl and season with the chicken seasoning. Drizzle the olive oil.

Use a spatula or your hands to coat well the chicken tenders on all sides.

Spray the air fryer basket with non-stick spray and place the chicken pieces in a single layer.

Cook for 10 minutes in the preheated air fryer and flip the tenders halfway.

Transfer to a plate and enjoy with your favorite sides.

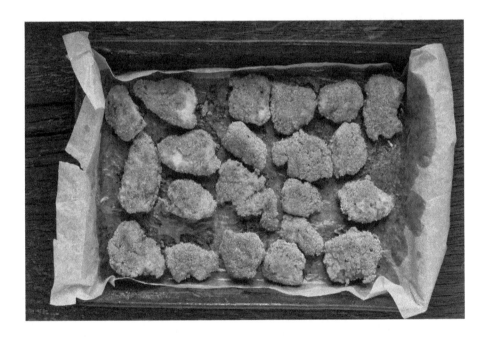

LIGHT CHICKEN AND VEGETABLES WITH AIR FRYER

Prep Time: 5 minutes Cook Time: 15 minutes0 minutes Total Time: 20 minutes Servings: 4 servings

Ingredients

1 pound chicken breast, chopped into bite-size pieces (2-3 medium chicken breasts)

1 cup broccoli florets (fresh or frozen)

1 zucchini chopped

1 cup bell pepper chopped (any colors you like)

1/2 onion chopped

2 clove garlic minced or crushed

2 tablespoons olive oil

1/2 teaspoon EACH garlic powder, chili powder, salt, pepper

1 tablespoon Italian seasoning (or spice blend of choice)

Instructions

Preheat air fryer to 400F.

Chop the veggies and chicken into small bite-size pieces and transfer to a large mixing bowl.

Add the oil and seasoning to the bowl and toss to combine.

Add the chicken and veggies to the preheated air fryer and cook for 10 minutes, shaking halfway, or until the chicken and veggies are charred and chicken is cooked through. If your air fryer is small, you may have to cook them in 2-3 batches.

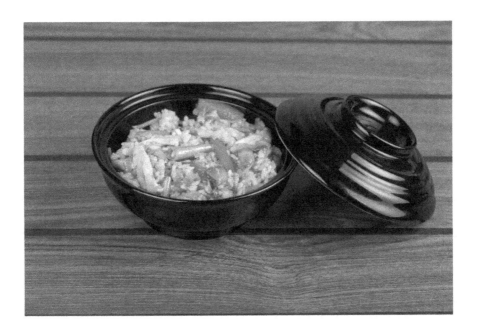

EXQUISITE VEGETABLES BROWNED WITH THE AIR FRYER

prep time: 10 MINUTES

cook time: 20 MINUTES

total time: 30 MINUTES

Ingredients

1 cup broccoli florets

1 cup cauliflower florets

1/2 cup baby carrots

1/2 cup yellow squash, sliced

1/2 cup baby zucchini, sliced

1/2 cup sliced mushrooms

1 small onion, sliced

1/4 cup balsamic vinegar

1 tablespoon olive oil

1 tablespoon minced garlic

1 teaspoon sea salt

1 teaspoon black pepper

1 teaspoon red pepper flakes

1/4 cup parmesan cheese

Instructions

Pre-heat Air Fryer at 400 for 3 minutes.

In a large bowl, put olive oil, balsamic vinegar, garlic, salt and pepper and red pepper flakes.

Super easy and delicious air fryer roasted vegetables that can be made super-fast for dinner in under 20 minutes! #healthyrecipe #vegetables #healthyeats

Whisk together.

Super easy and delicious air fryer roasted vegetables that can be made super-fast for dinner in under 20 minutes! #healthyrecipe #vegetables #healthyeats

Add vegetables and toss to coat.

Super easy and delicious air fryer roasted vegetables that can be made super-fast for dinner in under 20 minutes! #healthyrecipe #vegetables #healthyeats

Add vegetables to Air Fryer basket. Cook for 8 minutes.

Shake vegetables and cook for 6-8 additional minutes.

Super easy and delicious air fryer roasted vegetables that can be made super-fast for dinner in under 20 minutes! #healthyrecipe #vegetables #healthyeats

Add cheese and bake for 1-2 minutes.

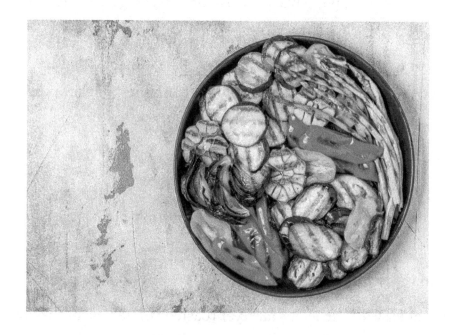

CHICKPEA & CARROT BALLS

Preparation Time: 5 minutes Cooking Time: 20 minutes
Servings: 3

Ingredients

2 tbsp. olive oil

2 tbsp. soy sauce

1 tbsp. flax meal

2 cups cooked chickpeas

½ cup sweet onions

½ cup grated carrots

½ cup roasted cashews

Juice of 1 lemon

½ tsp. turmeric

1 tsp. cumin

1 tsp. garlic powder

1 cup rolled oats

Instructions

Combine the olive oil, onions, and carrots into the Air Fryer baking pan and cook them on Air Fry function for 6 minutes at 350 F. Ground the oats and cashews in a food processor. Place in a large bowl. Mix in the chickpeas, lemon juice, and soy sauce.

Add onions and carrots to the bowl with chickpeas. Stir in the remaining ingredients; mix until fully incorporated. Make meatballs out of the mixture. Increase the temperature to 370 F and cook for 12 minutes.

EASY AIR FRYER TUNA STEAKS

YIELD: 2 SERVINGS

PREP TIME

20 minutes

COOK TIME

4 minutes

TOTAL TIME

24 minutes

Ingredients

2 (6 ounce) boneless and skinless yellowfin tuna steaks

1/4 cup soy sauce

2 teaspoons honey

1 teaspoon grated ginger

1 teaspoon sesame oil

1/2 teaspoon rice vinegar

OPTIONAL FOR SERVING

green onions, sliced

sesame seeds

Instructions

Remove the tuna steaks from the fridge.

In a large bowl, combine the soy sauce, honey, grated ginger, sesame oil, and rice vinegar.

Place tuna steaks in the marinade and let marinate for 20-30 minutes covered in the fridge.

Preheat air fryer to 380 degrees and then cook the tuna steaks in one layer for 4 minutes.

Let the air fryer tuna steaks rest for a minute or two, then slice, and enjoy immediately! Garnish with green onions and/or sesame seeds if desired

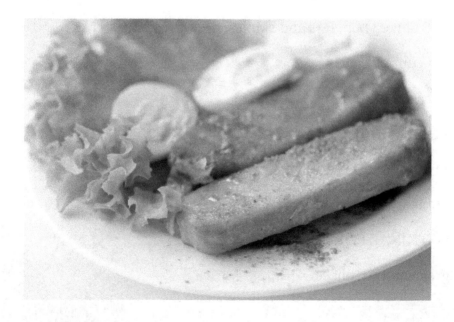

KETO AIR FRYER GARLIC CHICKEN BREAST

YIELD: 4 SERVINGS

PREP TIME

2 minutes

COOK TIME

10 minutes

TOTAL TIME

12 minutes

Ingredients

4 boneless chicken breasts

2 tablespoons butter

1/4 teaspoon garlic powder

1/2 teaspoon salt

1/4 teaspoon pepper

Instructions

Place boneless chicken breasts on a cutting board.

Melt butter in the microwave and add in garlic powder, salt, and pepper. Mix to combine.

Coat chicken with butter mixture on both sides.

Place chicken in the air fryer in one single layer.

Cook chicken at 380 degrees for 10-15 minutes, flipping halfway. The chicken is done once the chicken reads 165 degrees at its thickest part.

Let chicken rest for 5 minutes.

Enjoy immediately or refrigerate and enjoy cold or using reheated directions above.

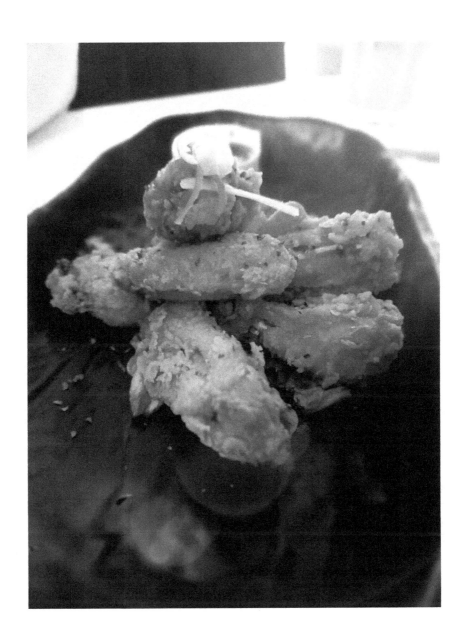

RIBEYE STEAK FRIES

YIELD: 2 SERVINGS

PREP TIME

5 minutes

COOK TIME

10 minutes

ADDITIONAL TIME

30 minutes

TOTAL TIME

45 minutes

Ingredients

8-ounce ribeye steak, about 1-inch thick

1 tablespoon McCormick Montreal Steak Seasoning

Instructions

Remove the ribeye steak from the fridge and season with the Montreal Steak seasoning. Let steak rest for about 20 minutes to come to room temperature (to get a more tender juicy steak).

Preheat your air fryer to 400 degrees.

Place the ribeye steak in the air fryer and cook for 10-12 minutes, until it reaches 130-135 degrees for medium rare. Cook for an additional 5 minutes for medium-well.

Remove the steak from the air fryer and let rest at least 5 minutes before cutting to keep the juices inside the steak then enjoy!

How to preheat steak in the air fryer:

1. Preheat your air fryer to 350 degrees.

2. Cook steak in the air fryer for 3 to 5 minutes until heated thoroughly, let sit fot 5 minutes, then enjoy!

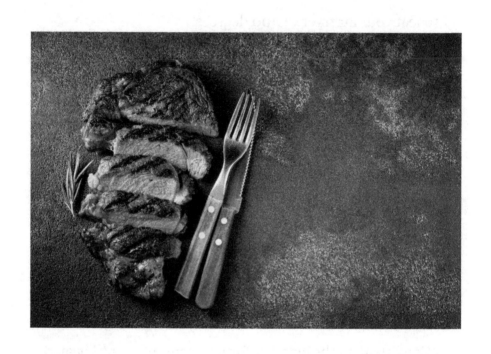

SAUSAGE BREAKFAST PATTIES

YIELD: 4 SERVINGS

COOK TIME

6 minutes

TOTAL TIME

6 minutes

Ingredients

8 raw sausage breakfast Pattie

Instructions

Preheat your air fryer to 370 degrees.

Place the raw sausage patties in the air fryer in one layer not touching.

Cook for 6-8 minutes, until they reach 160 degrees. *

Remove from the air fryer and enjoy!

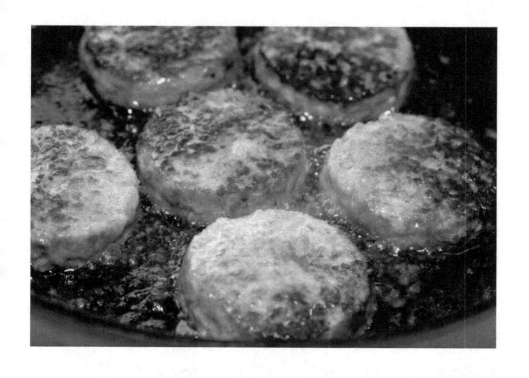